Medicinal Herbs

A Beginner's Guide

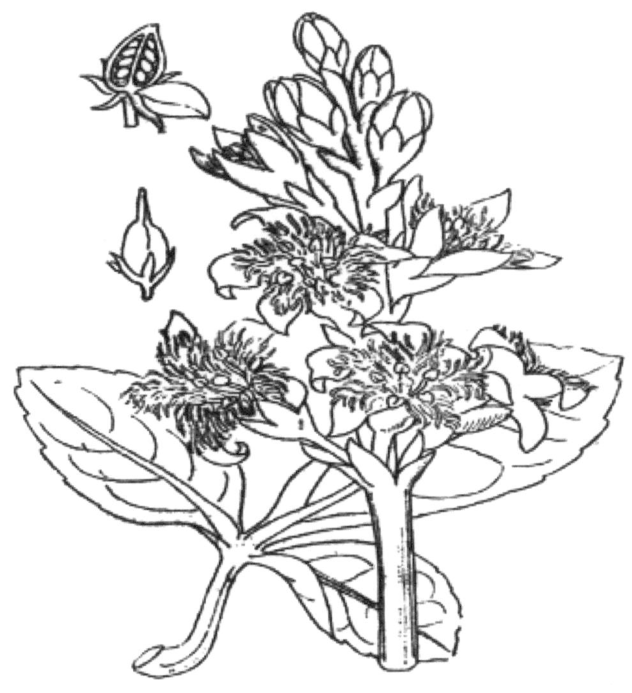

Martin Pals

Table of Contents

Introduction

Congratulations on downloading *Medicinal Herbs: A Beginner's Guide* and thank you for doing so. While a shift towards natural wellness has been a popular trend over the last few years, the use of herbs in medicine actually dates back to 1500 BC. The ancient Egyptians wrote a lengthy scroll document detailing hundreds of medicinal herbal remedies. Herbs also played a significant role in the Middle Ages and were a medical staple for Native Americans.

Unfortunately, during the 1900s scientific advancements pushed herbs out of the medical community. Doctors preferred using chemical, man-made medicines to herbs. The power and potency of natural remedies began being questioned, mocked, and shunned by medical institutions. Instead of using herbs, doctors and hospitals started administering pharmaceuticals to treat patients. They no longer believed in the healing power of plants.

Luckily the rise of the Internet has empowered people all over the world to easily learn about homeopathic and alternative medicines. We now can do research for ourselves and learn about natural healing. Herbs are on the rise again and can be conveniently purchased online, at health food stores, and even traditional pharmacies and grocery chains have jumped on the bandwagon and begun carrying herb supplements. In today's eBook, we'll be going over a few of the most well-known herbs. You'll learn about their uses, benefits of consumption, and how you can even grow them on your own. We think you'll be surprised to learn about the many wonderful powers these herbs have, and how simple it truly is to consume them in your daily life.

Chapter 1: Echinacea

What is Echinacea?

If you've ever shopped at a health food store, you've probably seen Echinacea supplements. Echinacea is a perennial in the daisy family and grows in North and Central America. It can grow in moist or dry climates.

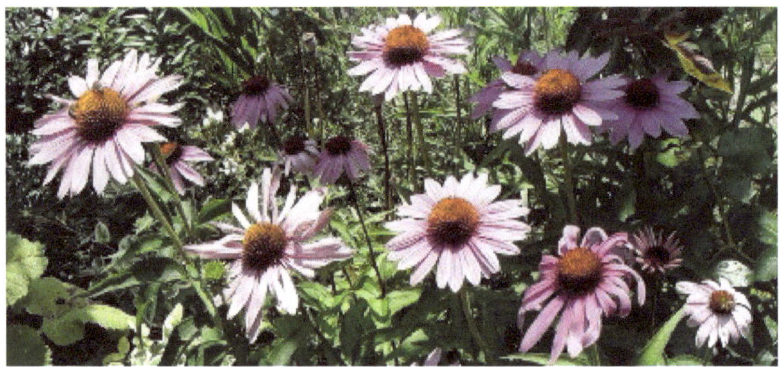

Echinacea purpurea, purple coneflower

Benefits of Echinacea

Echinacea is an immune system powerhouse, which is why it's such a well-known herb and so heavily consumed. It's excellent for the immune system because it can help increase production of white blood cells. This is important because white blood cells are part of our bodies' immune systems and help protect our bodies from viruses. When we don't produce enough white blood cells, and our counts are low, we're more susceptible to catching an illness.

Taking Echinacea regularly can strengthen your immune system significantly, making you feel healthy and strong every day and also prevent you from catching strep throat, or whatever stomach bug or cold that's going around. Herbalists recommend consuming Echinacea during flu season or before going someplace where you'll be exposed to a high number of germs, such as airports, planes, buses, and trains. Many people take it at the first sign of cold and flu symptoms to keep themselves from getting sick. Echinacea can also be consumed while you're sick to help speed up your recovery time so that you start to feel better faster. Echinacea also has anti-bacterial properties, which make it effective for treating fungal and bacterial infections. This also makes it useful for healing wounds and yeast infection relief. Some even use Echinacea to treat upset stomach, diarrhea, and indigestion and find that it works better than over the counter medicines.

Consuming and Using Echinacea

Echinacea is most commonly consumed in a pill form. Most natural food stores, conventional supermarkets, and drugstores carry Echinacea supplement capsules. This is probably the easiest way to consume it. You can also find Echinacea teas online or at your favorite health food store. Echinacea tea is just as effective as the pills. It typically has a floral taste, but some teas combine it with other herbs to make it more palatable. Additionally, it also comes in a liquid form, which is recommended for those using Echinacea to treat tonsillitis or strep throat. The liquid can also be applied to cuts and fungal infections on the skin. Liquid Echinacea can be easily found online, in natural markets, grocery stores, and big-box retailers like Target and Wal-Mart.

Growing Echinacea

Aside from being an amazing antifungal, antibiotic, and immune system supplement, Echinacea is also a beautiful flower! You'll love growing it for both its healing abilities and the beauty its bright purple petals will add to your herb garden. In bloom, Echinacea looks like just a standard daisy, but with purple petals instead of white. These lovely perennials bloom throughout summer and fall.

For starters, make sure to plant Echinacea where it will receive plenty of sunlight. It grows best with full sun but can bloom with partial shade. It's best to plant your Echinacea plant in the fall or in the early spring. With seeds, the ideal time to sow is early springtime as the seeds need to be cold to germinate. They can grow to be fairly big, so it's recommended to leave about a foot and a half between each plant. As a plant, Echinacea isn't very picky about the soil in which it's planted. Some people can grow Echinacea without any problem in poor soil or in soil with lots of rocks. However, to be safe, it's best to use rich soil free of rocks.

Another great thing about growing Echinacea is that it doesn't require a lot of watering, making it an ideal herb to grow if you live in a drier climate, or if you're not the best at remembering to water your plants. During the plant's infancy, it's important to water it daily or every other day. As your Echinacea plant grows, you'll get away with watering it just twice a week. In full bloom, you can water it as little as weekly or every other week. If you live in a climate that gets adequate rain, you can stop watering it yourself and let Mother Nature handle it. In climates that do receive rain, you don't have to water it after the second year.

 Most people consume their own Echinacea by making a tea out of the leaves and petals. To do this, pluck them soon after the plant has bloomed. Rinse the petals and leaves with water, and then let them dry. When they've fully dried, you can steep them in hot water. After steeping, use a strainer to filter out the dried petals and leaves and then you can consume the tea. Some people prefer to make tea out of the root and believe that the root is more potent. This is fine to do, but be sure you don't cut the entire root so that the plant can grow again. If you choose to do this, make sure to do it later in the fall after the flowers have bloomed. Rinse the root, finely chop it, and then allow it to air dry. Steep it in hot water and strain before drinking. Whether you make the tea from petals, leaves, or roots (or a combination of the three) is up to you.

Chapter 2: St. John's Wort

What is St. John's Wort?

Hypericum perforatum, better known as St. John's Wort, is a yellow perennial flower that's often mistaken for a weed. You may have heard of it if you or a loved one has suffered from mild to moderate depression.

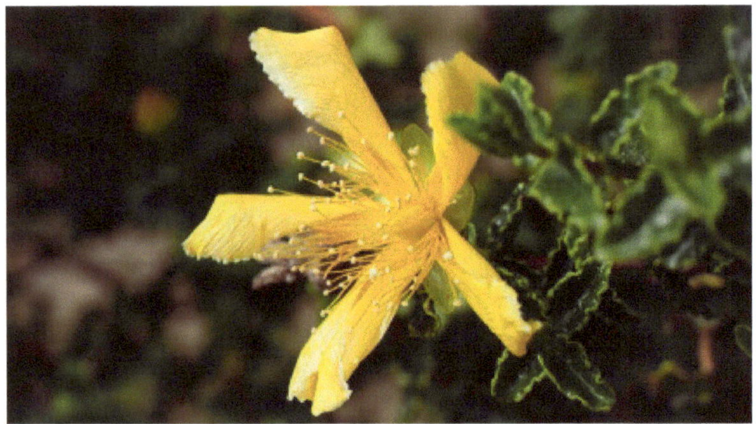

St John'S Wort Blossom Bloom

Benefits of St. John's Wort

St. John's Wort is often used to treat depression, general anxiety, premenstrual syndrome, social anxiety, chronic fatigue, and seasonal depression. Some studies have found that it's just as effective, or even more effective, at treating these conditions than prescription antidepressants. It's believed that St.

John's Wort can increase serotonin, noradrenaline, and dopamine levels, which makes it useful for those suffering from mood disorders. When those chemical levels are low, people may experience anxiety and depression symptoms such as nervousness, hopelessness, insomnia, fatigue, decreased appetite, low libido, and poor concentration. As you can imagine, these feelings are unpleasant and can interrupt one's life. This is why many people who struggle with anxiety and depression seek some type of medical treatment. Since depression can be a serious illness and can greatly impact your life and overall health, St. John's Wort is typically not used for more severe cases. Generally, it's only recommended for mild to moderate cases of depression or anxiety-related disorders. If you're suffering from depression or anxiety related condition, you should consult your doctor before taking St. John's Wort as it can have an adverse reaction when taken in conjunction with other medications.

St. John's Wort can be a natural alternative to chemical medications such as selective serotonin reuptake inhibitors (SSRIs) for mental health issues. Some people don't like the idea of taking an SSRI and prefer to only use natural treatments, which is why they turn to St. John's Wort. Anxiety can really throw your hormones out of whack, and St. John's Wort can help reset you. It can regulate your stress hormones, which helps with common anxiety symptoms such as insomnia, fatigue, and mood swings. In fact, it's so good at treating mood swings and hormonal issues that it's often recommended to women who struggle with a severe premenstrual syndrome. Some women find that the hormonal changes that occur during menopause worsen their mood, decrease their libido, and cause lethargy. St. John's Wort can alleviate these symptoms in menopausal women. Lesser-known benefits of St. John's Wort are that it has strong anti-inflammatory and antibacterial properties. This makes it helpful for treating wounds, burns, hemorrhoids, and eczema.

Consuming and Using St. John's Wort

St. John's Wort is sold in capsule form, and this is how it's consumed for treating mood and mental health issues. There's also a liquid form that you can take if you prefer that over pills. You can find St. John's Wort capsules and liquids online, at health food stores, and sometimes in drugstores. Dosage varies based on the condition you're treating, which is why you should always following the pills' instructions on how to consume them. You should also speak with a doctor, naturopath, or herbalist to see if you're a good candidate for taking St. John's Wort and for determining the dosage. For treating skin issues, St. John's Wort is sold in tincture and lotion form to be applied topically. Not all health food stores carry St. John's Wort in these forms, but they're easy to find online. For aiding eczema, wounds, and burns, apply the tincture or the lotion to the affected area on your skin. Again, follow instructions and speak to a professional about how much to apply and how often.

Growing St. John's Wort

What's lovely about St. John's Wort is that it has a bright yellow flower. This makes it a cheerful and bright addition to your garden, which is fitting since it's used for treating anxiety and depression. The seeds need to be planted after the frost has passed, and should be placed where they'll receive full sun or partial shade since they really need plenty of sunshine to germinate. You could also plant your seeds indoors, so long as you do so a few weeks before frost. If you do this, make sure to keep them near a window or skylight so that they can germinate. During germination, water as often as needed to keep the soil moist. After that, water weekly or as needed.

Many people like to use St. John's Wort to make their own tea. As a tea, St. John's Wort has a mild lemony flavor. To make tea, cut the flowers when your St. John's Wort is in full bloom (typically mid-summer). Gently rinse the flowers with cold water and then steep them in hot water for a few minutes. Strain the flowers out before drinking. To treat skin conditions such as cuts, burns, and eczema, you can use St. John's Wort flowers to make a healing oil. For maximum potency, pluck the buds from your flowers right before they're about to bloom. Place the buds in a canning car. Fill the jar with an oil of your choosing, such as jojoba oil or olive oil, so that the buds are completely submerged. It's important for the buds to be covered by the oil so that they won't grow mold. Seal the jar and let it sit on a windowsill where it will receive plenty of light. Check the jar daily, and if you notice any condensation forming, you should open the jar and wipe it out. After three or four weeks, you'll see that the oil/bud concoction has turned dark red – this is how you'll know that it's ready for use. Strain the buds out of the oil and then store it in a small, tight container. Apply the oil to infected areas on your skin. Depending on the severity of your skin condition, it can take a few days or weeks to see results.

Chapter 3: Chamomile

What is Chamomile?

Chances are you've tried chamomile tea at least once in your life. In fact, we're willing to bet that you may have a box of it somewhere in your cupboard. Chamomile tea is one of the most popular types of tea because of it's sweet, floral taste and also because it's naturally caffeine free. What you may not have known is that chamomile is part of the daisy family and drinking it has several health benefits. If you're already a chamomile tea drinker, you'll be happy to learn what this herb can do for your health and how easy it is to grow it yourself.

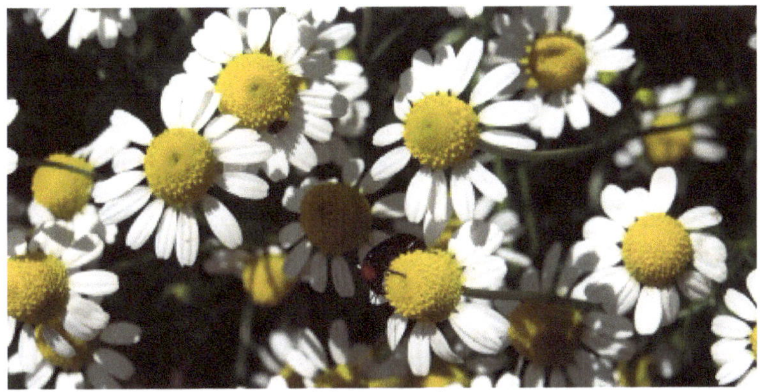
Chamomile

Benefits of Chamomile

Chamomile tea is commonly used as a sleep aid. The chamomile plant naturally contains the antioxidant apigenin, which acts as a mild tranquilizer and induces sleepiness. People who suffer from insomnia are often able to get themselves to sleep by drinking a cup of chamomile tea before bedtime. Not only does it help you feel drowsy at bedtime, but it can also improve the quality of your sleep, which makes it useful for people who find that they suffer from poor-quality sleep. The apigenin in chamomile can also bring relief to people who are stressed or who struggle with anxiety. If you feel anxious or are going through a particularly stressful time in your life, you may be able to unwind by drinking chamomile tea regularly. People under stress and who have general anxiety often find that simply drinking a cup of this tea helps improve their mood and also helps them feel more calm and relaxed.

Apigenin is also believed to play a role in fighting and preventing the growth of certain cancer cells. Studies have found that apigenin can help prevent breast, prostate, and uterine cancers. In addition to apigenin, chamomile is chockfull of flavone antioxidants. Flavones can lower cholesterol and blood pressure levels, which promotes better heart health. Some studies have found that drinking chamomile tea regularly can significantly improve your heart's health.

Chamomile also has anti-inflammatory properties, which make it useful for improving digestion, treating gas, and soothing an upset stomach. Because of this, many people drink a cup of chamomile tea after a meal or if they're experiencing any type of digestive discomfort. Some people even find that it brings them relief if they have diarrhea.

Consuming and Using Chamomile

Of course, chamomile is most commonly used for tea. You can find chamomile tea virtually anywhere – grocery stores, online, big-box retailers, drugstores, and natural food stores. Drinking it as a tea is the best way to treat sleeplessness, anxiety, stress, diarrhea, gas, and upset stomach. It's also the best way to use chamomile for improving heart health. However, if you're not a tea drinker you can also take it in a capsule form if you want to use chamomile for digestive purposes or to treat anxiousness and insomnia.

Aside from consuming chamomile as a tea or pill supplement, you can also take advantage of its healing properties as an essential oil. Applied topically, chamomile oil can fight bacterial and fungal infections, heal cuts, treat acne, and stimulate circulation. You can also simply smell the oil or put it in an essential oil diffuser to improve your mood if you're feeling sad or anxious. Inhaling the oil can even ease nausea and improve digestion. You can find chamomile oil online and at many health food stores.

Growing Chamomile

Chamomile is relatively easy to grow and tends to grow best in cooler conditions with some shade, although it can grow in full sun. It's a low maintenance herb and won't need watering once it's established as long as you live in a climate that gets some rain. If you live in an area prone to drought, you will need to monitor it and water it as needed.

To make tea, cut flowers from your chamomile. You don't want too much of the flower stems or too many leaves, as they'll affect the flavor. Rinse the flowers and then steep them in hot water, and then strain before drinking. For best flavor, cut the flowers the same day you plan on having the tea.

To make your own chamomile essential oil, pluck chamomile flowers from your plant. Rinse them and allow them to dry before placing them in a canning jar. Fill the jar with olive oil so that the flowers are completely submerged. Seal the jar and let it somewhere where it will receive several hours of sunlight each day. Check on it regularly and if you see condensation forming, be sure to wipe it. After two or three weeks, strain the oil. You can then use it for aromatherapy or applying topically. For maximum results, try drinking your chamomile tea while smelling the oil or applying it to your body. You may find that using the oil and tea together amplifies the results and promotes even more feelings of tranquility.

Chapter 4: Lavender

What is Lavender?

If you've studied aromatherapy or if you enjoy gardening, you've probably seen and smelled Lavendula, better known as lavender. Most people love lavender's scent, which is why it's commonly used in floral arrangements, air sprays, lotions, soaps, candles, and perfumes. Some people even like baking with lavender and putting it in lemonade or cocktails to enjoy its sweet, floral taste. There's a reason why lavender is so popular, and here we'll explain why lavender is such an amazing herb.

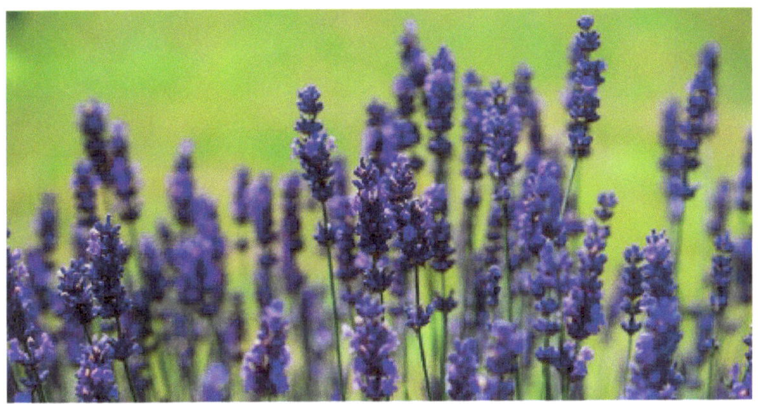

Lavender

Benefits of Lavender

Lavender oil can help reduce stress and improve your mood in many ways. For one, smelling lavender or consuming it in a capsule form can help treat anxiety and depression. Some herbalists and naturopaths even recommend it to patients suffering from posttraumatic stress disorder (PTSD) and post-partum depression. They find that lavender can help people feel relax, prevent moodiness and mood swings. Some people suffer from insomnia or poor quality sleep if they're experiencing anxiety or depression. Supplementing with lavender or using it for aromatherapy can help promote sleep and help people stay asleep throughout the night. Even if you don't have a serious case of anxiety, you still may find that diffusing lavender oil in your bedroom before you go to sleep helps you feel more relax and fall asleep faster.

Lavender can also be used for pain relief. People suffering from migraines, tension headaches, and menstrual cramps find that lavender can help ease their pain. Simply inhaling lavender can significantly decrease the excruciating pain experienced during a migraine or regular tension headache. Some people find that they're able to minimize their headache pain by applying the oil to their temple, shoulders, or back of the neck. For menstrual cramps, massaging the abdomen with lavender oil can help alleviate the pain. If you're sore or experience joint pain, you can apply lavender oil to the areas in pain on your body and may find that the pain subsides.

In addition to pain relief, lavender oil aromatherapy can be a great tool for cancer patients. Not only does the scent of lavender help improve one's mood, which is important for cancer patients since many suffer from depression and anxiety after receiving their diagnosis, but it can also boost their weakened immune systems. Cancer treatments such as chemotherapy can deplete the immune system, and boosting it back up with lavender is a good way for cancer patients to start to build up their health. Many cancer patients struggle with sleeping due to pain and discomfort, and applying lavender oil topically can reduce pain and help promote sleep so that cancer patients can get the rest that their bodies need.

Lavender has antioxidants and anti-inflammatory properties, which makes it great for skin and hair. It can heal fungal and bacterial skin infections and rashes, as well as burns, cuts, and canker sores. The antioxidants make it great for anti-aging by preventing wrinkles, strengthening your skin's elasticity, and giving skin an overall glow.

Consuming and Using Lavender

To use lavender essential oil to practice aromatherapy, you can buy it at health food stores, specialty shops, and online. You can then apply the oil to your skin, sniff it from the bottle, or put it in an air diffuser. People using lavender for pain relief would inhale it or apply it to the skin as well. As mentioned previously, lavender is also sold in a capsule form. People who are sensitive to smell or who want to take advantage of lavender's healing powers without aromatherapy can start by capsules online or at natural herb and supplement stores. Often times people choose to take the supplements to use lavender to treat sleep issues, improve mood, and to promote calmness.

And of course, lavender oil can be a cheap alternative to expensive perfumes. Put a few drops on your wrists, décolletage, and behind your ears to give yourself a nice lavender scent. You can also mix it into your favorite non-scented lotion and hand cream. If you practice soap making, you can add it to your handmade soaps.

Growing Lavender

Lavender is a beautiful flower that adds a pop of color to your garden. It also smells wonderful, and as you now know, it boasts multiple medicinal benefits. It only makes sense that you would want to grow this amazing herb. Plant your lavender about a foot and a half apart to give it plenty of room. The soil should be well drained, and it should be an area that receives plenty of sunlight. Be careful not to overwater your plants, and remember that they don't need daily water. Only water your lavender when the soil is completely dry. As your lavender grows, you may find that you don't need to water it at all – it really depends on the climate in which you live.

To make lavender oil, cut a few sprigs of lavender. Chop off the long stems, as you only want to be working with the flowers and the stems near the base of the flowers. Wrap the sprigs in a thin cloth, tying them tightly with a string or rubber band. Hang the wrapped springs upside in a dry, warm area for about

two weeks. Avoid direct sunlight as it might break
down the oils. After the lavender has dried, crumble it
into small pieces. Pour the dried lavender crumbles
into a canning jar and submerge them with oil. We
recommend almond oil or jojoba oil, as you don't want
to use something that will overpower the lavender's
aroma. Seal the jar and place it in sunlight. You can
open the jar in as little as two days, but if you want a
stronger fragrance, you should wait two weeks.
Strain the lavender out of the oil. You can then use
the oil for topical skincare treatments and
aromatherapy.

Chapter 5: Marigold

What is Marigold?

Marigold is a bright, golden colored flower that you've probably seen in floral arrangements and gardens. Perhaps you even have marigolds growing in your yard! They're a well-known flower that most people can recognize and identify, even if they know little about gardening and flowers. However, not nearly as many people know that these flowers also have healing properties. In fact, Calendula officinalis (one type of marigold) has been used for healing dating back to the eleventh and twelfth centuries.

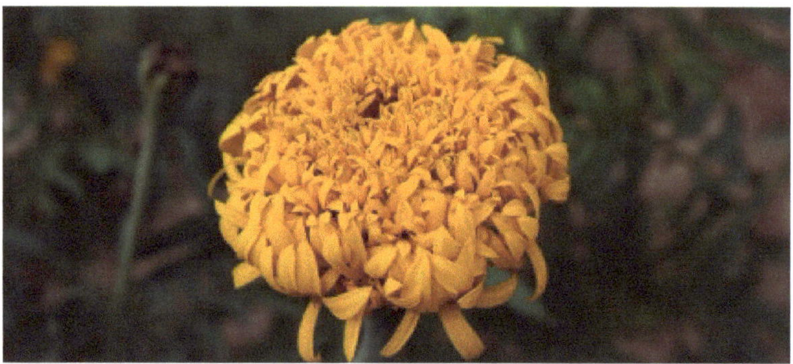

Marigold flower

Benefits of Marigold

Marigold contains antioxidants, which make it a multi-purpose herb that can be used in numerous ways. For one, these antioxidants make it great for the immune system. Naturopaths often have sick patients take marigold to ease common cold and flu symptoms, such as sore throat, fever, and cough. Marigold can also be taken preventatively to keep your immune system strong during cold and flu season, and before traveling. If you've ever used an anti-aging product, you've probably seen that many claims to have antioxidants. This is because antioxidants fight free radicals, which attack the skin's barrier and leave skin looking sagging, wrinkled, dull, and discolored. The antioxidants in marigold make it great for anti-aging by fighting free radical damage and keeping skin firm, smooth, and bright for a healthy, youthful appearance. Additionally, if you suffer from acne, you may find that the antioxidants in marigold reduce the inflammation from your blemishes. Marigold also contains antiseptic properties, which help treat acne caused by bacteria on the skin and can help treat fungal skin infections and cuts.

The anti-inflammatory property of marigold makes it effective for digestive issues. People who suffer from acid reflux, gastritis, inflammatory bowel disease, and stomach cramps may find that marigold eases their pain and helps them manage their symptoms. Marigold can also improve blood flow circulation, making it helpful for people experiencing muscle spasms or cramps. It helps blood flow to the cramped area, therefore subduing the pain and stopping the body's inflammatory response.

Another important benefit of marigolds is their ability to ward off bugs. You may have already known this if you've purchased holistic bug spray. If you live in a humid climate with lots of mosquitoes you probably have to deal with irritating bug bites. Marigold's scent is a natural repellent that can help keep you safe from mosquitoes.

Consuming and Using Marigold

To take advantage of marigold's ability to support the immune and digestive systems, many people drink marigold tea. This tea can be found at most grocery stores and organic food markets. For cold and flu symptom relief, you can swallow a few drops of marigold extract. These drops can be found at health food stores, online, and in Ayurvedic clinics and stores. To treat skin conditions and to take advantage of marigold's antioxidants, you can apply salves, creams, and ointments made from marigold. You can also just apply the marigold oil to areas on your skin that have rashes or infections to help clear them up, reduce inflammation, and stop the itching.

As mentioned earlier, marigolds can be used to keep bugs at bay. Apply marigold oil to your skin before going outside to prevent mosquito bites. You may also find that lighting marigold scented candles outside can make your backyard less buggy. For gardeners, planting marigold in the garden can protect your other plants from being eaten by microscopic worms, aphids, and other bugs.

Growing Marigold

Begin by planting your seeds indoors in pots. You should do this a month and a half or two months before the last frost date. Cover the pot with saran wrap and leave it in a dry, dark place. Marigolds don't need any light until they germinate, so they should be left in the dark during this time. After three or four days, you'll find that the seeds have germinated. If you live in a cooler environment, it may take a few more days. When you see that they've germinated, you can remove the saran wrap and move them into direct sunlight. At this point, they'll need at least five hours a day of light. Keep the potting soil moist so that the seeds can continue to grow. When the seedlings start to grow a few leaves you can plant them outdoors. Once outside, you can stop watering them. If you live in a dry climate that receives little rain, you'll need to give them a bit of water every two weeks.

Once your marigold plants have bloomed, you can use their flowers to make healing tea. Harvest a few flowers, pull apart the petals and lay them out to dry for a few days. Check on them to make sure that they've completely dried, and then you can steep them in hot water. To create marigold infused oil, follow the same process of drying out marigold petals. Once fully dried, put the petals in a canning jar. Fill the jar with olive oil, jojoba oil, or almond oil so that the petals are all completely submerged. Seal the jar tightly and leave it on a windowsill or somewhere you know it will get plenty of light. Check on it every day to make sure that condensation isn't forming, and if

you do see any open the jar to clean it away. After
about four weeks you can strain the oil and then start
applying it topically to your skin.

Chapter 6: Peppermint

What is Peppermint?

We're sure that you know what peppermint is, and that at some point in your life you've had peppermint-flavored gum, candy, chocolates, or tea. You're probably familiar with its taste and color, but you may not know that it has been a part of naturopathic medicine for centuries. Aside from its delicious taste that you associate with some of your favorite sweets, this herb has many healing properties that you can easily take advantage of.

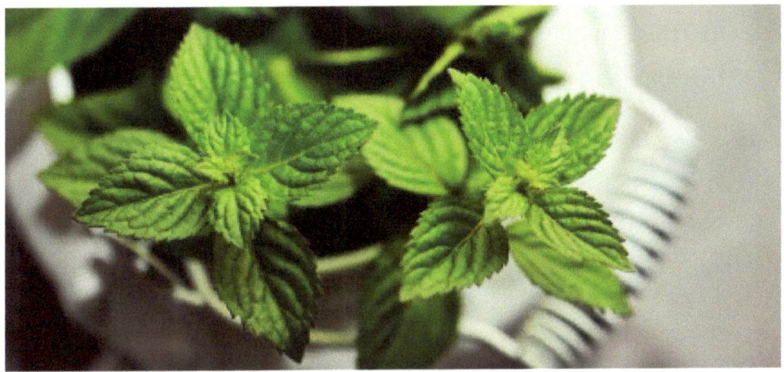

Peppermint

Benefits of Peppermint

Peppermint can treat numerous digestive issues. It can provide relief to people suffering from irritable bowel syndrome, indigestion, and gas. It can relax your intestinal muscles, allowing gas and waste to pass through more easily and therefore reducing abdominal discomfort. Drinking peppermint tea can help ease an upset stomach. Aside from helping your digestive tract, peppermint can improve your respiratory system. If your sinus and lungs are congested when you're sick, inhaling peppermint oil or massaging it on your chest can help decongest you. The rosmarinic acid naturally found in peppermint can also help reduce inflammation in people with asthma.

Like many other medicinal herbs, peppermint can be used for pain relief. Inhaling peppermint oil or applying it to the temple, wrists, and forehead and be helpful in alleviating tension headache pain. The oil can also be massaged into sore muscles and joints. If you're sore all over, you can soak in a bath with some peppermint oil. You could also do this if you're under stress, as peppermint's aroma can help make people feel more calm and relaxed.

You've probably noticed that many gums, mouthwashes, and toothpaste are peppermint flavored. This isn't just because of its nice taste. Peppermint can freshen breath and help prevent the formation of cavities because of its antimicrobial properties. These properties along with its anti-inflammatory properties also make it effective for treating acne, psoriasis, and eczema.

Consuming and Using Peppermint

The best way to use peppermint to treat digestive issues is to drink it in tea form. Peppermint tea is easy to find and is sold virtually everywhere that tea is sold. It's a popular tea because of its nice flavor, and most people enjoy. For aromatherapy and applying it topically for skin issues and pain relief, you can find peppermint oil at health food stores, online, and in alternative medicine stores. You can use the oil in a diffuse, sniff it out of the bottle, or apply it to a cloth and then inhale it. For topical application, simply rub it into the area of your skin that you wish to treat.

For oral health, you can use peppermint oil to make your own mouthwash and toothpaste. Before ingesting it or putting it into your mouth, make sure that the oil is high quality and can be consumed.

Growing Peppermint

Plant peppermint in a moist site where it will receive adequate light. These plants can survive with some shade, but they do need to get enough sunlight each day. Plant seeds about two feet apart because its known to spread a decent amount as it grows. Your peppermint plants will need about an inch of water each week, so you may not even have to water them depending on where you live.

To make tea, pick five to ten leaves from your peppermint plant. Make sure that they look green and healthy, and that they haven't been bitten by any bugs. Rinse the leaves and then crush them into small bits. Add them to your tea mug, and then fill it with hot water. After a few minutes, you can strain

the leaves out of the tea. You can steep it longer if
you want a stronger flavor.

To make essential oil, wash and crush freshly picked
peppermint leaves. Lay the leaves out to dry and
allow them to dry completely. Once dry, crumble the
dried leaves and put them in a canning jar. Fill the jar
with jojoba or almond oil so that the leaves are
completely submerged. If leaves float to the surface,
give the jar a light shake and then add a little more oil.
Seal the jar tightly and let it sit overnight in a cool,
dark place. After twenty-four hours have passed,
open the jar and strain out the leaves. Pick more
fresh peppermint leaves. Wash, dry, and crumble the
leaves and add them to the jar of oil. You may need
to add a bit more oil to keep the new leaves
submerged. Allow the jar to sit overnight and then
strain after twenty-four hours. You can then use the
oil, or repeat the process a few more times if you want
a stronger smelling oil.

Chapter 7: Holy Basil

What is Holy Basil?

If you follow wellness trends, you may have heard about adaptogenic herbs. Right now, "adaptogen" is the latest natural health and wellness buzzword. Adaptogens are natural, plant-based substances that help the body cope with stress and help the physiology function normally. Holy basil is just one of many adaptogenic herbs, and it supplementing it can have numerous health benefits.

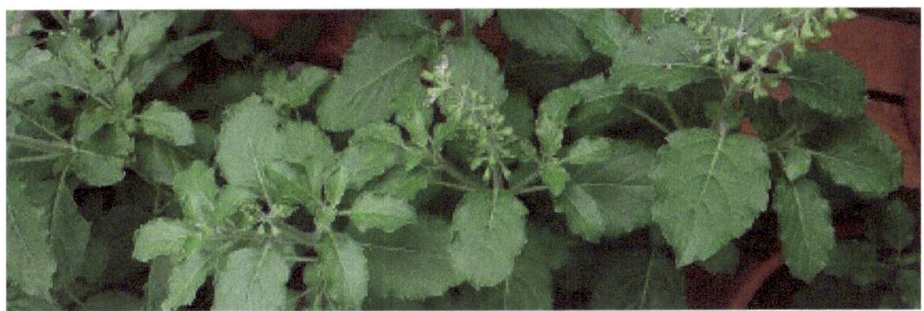

Holy Basil

Benefits of Holy Basil

Holy basil is best known for managing cortisol. Cortisol is an adrenal stress hormone that we secrete when we're stressed, scared, or going into what's often referred to as "fight or flight." While this sounds like a bad thing, the reality is that we *need* cortisol. It's what gives us a boost of power when we're exercising, and we need it during important moments in which we need to have energy and be alert. Our cortisol levels are supposed to change throughout the day - with higher levels in the morning so that we can wake up and start our days, and lower levels at night so we can relax and fall asleep. Thanks to the endless stressors of today's modern life, many people have cortisol levels that are alarmingly high. Similarly, many of us have our levels out of whack where we're producing too much cortisol at night and not enough during the day, causing us to stay up late at night and feel sluggish during daytime hours. Other unpleasant side effects of high cortisol levels include weight gain, constipation, weakened immune system, fatigue, infertility, insomnia, acne, and increased blood pressure. Cortisol is an important hormone that we need in our bodies, but we need the levels to be right. Otherwise, it will wreak havoc on our bodies.

As an adaptogen, holy basil can help restore cortisol levels to what they should be. Taken over time, holy basil will help you feel more relaxed and able to cope with your day-to-day stress. No more finding yourself in a full-blown panic over normal things that typically wouldn't bother you. Holy basil will also reset your internal clock so that your cortisol levels are high when you need them to be (in the morning and throughout the day) and then decrease in the evening so that you're able to fall asleep at a reasonable hour each night.

Aside from stress relief, holy basil can also prevent cancer. Some studies have found that people who take holy basil are less likely to develop cancer cells. For people who already have cancer, holy basil can fight against existing cancer cells and prevent new ones from growing and spreading. Holy basil is an antimicrobial herb, which makes it good for treating acne. Consuming it in capsule form and applying it topically can help reduce the number of breakouts and clear up existing blemishes.

In addition to being good for the skin, holy basil is also good for your bones, heart, and respiratory system. Holy basil has Vitamin K, and many people are deficient in it. This vitamin can help strengthen bone density, which is especially important for people as they age. Vitamin K is also good for keeping your heart healthy and strong. People with respiratory problems such as asthma often find that holy basil helps them breathe easier.

Consuming and Using Holy Basil

Most people who use holy basil take it as a supplement. Holy basil pills can be found at most health food stores, natural vitamin shops, and of course online. Supplements are best for people who are taking holy basil to regulate cortisol levels, prevent and treat cancer, and care for bone health, the heart, and respiratory system. Fewer people know that holy basil essential oil can be great for the body. Holy basil works wonders for aromatherapy and can help decrease anxiety. If you suffer from high cortisol levels or levels that are out of whack, taking a holy basil supplement in conjunction with diffusing the oil can be very effective. For treating acne, you can apply the oil to breakouts. Holy basil oil can be found online and in certain health food stores.

Growing Holy Basil

You can plant holy basil seeds in your garden after the last springtime frost. Be sure to plant them in an area where they'll receive at least five or six hours of direct sunlight each day. Water them lightly so that the soil and plants are moist, but be sure not to over water them. One thing you need to know is that you should harvest all of the holy basil plants before the autumnal frost. After the frost, they'll die, and you'll be left with mushy plants.

When your plants have grown leaves, you can make an essential oil by harvesting a few bunches of leaves. Wash and dry the leaves, and when they're completely dry, you can grind them until they form a paste. Mix the paste and half a cup of organic coconut oil, and heat them in a pot on low heat. After the paste and oil have mixed, cool the mixture and then store it in an airtight container. You can now use it topically and for aromatherapy.

Chapter 8: Rosemary

What is Rosemary?

You probably have tasted and smelled rosemary if you cook or have ever eaten Mediterranean, Spanish, or French cuisine. Aside from being a tasty seasoning for cooking, rosemary has been known to have several health benefits that are lesser known. The more you learn about what rosemary can do for your health, the more you'll want to cook with it.

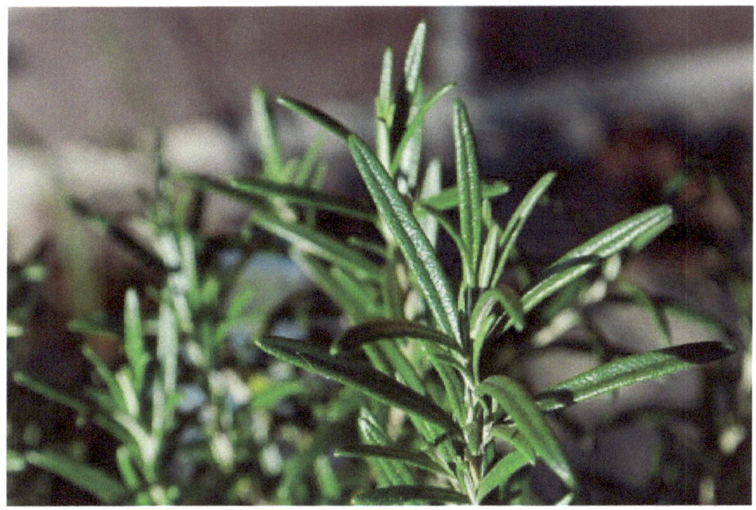

Rosemary

Benefits of Rosemary

Many people believe that rosemary is good for the brain. Several studies have found that it's a cognitive

39

stimulant and can help you with focus and even boosting overall intelligence. Because of this, people have started studying rosemary to see how it can help with memory retention. Some researchers have found that rosemary can help improve memory in people with dementia and Alzheimer's disease. In addition to helping your brain, rosemary can also be great for your mood. Its scent can help relieve stress, boost mood, and calm people with anxiety. When eaten, rosemary can have the same soothing effects.

Rosemary's anti-inflammatory and antibacterial properties also make it great for treating stomach issues. It can help fight and prevent bacterial stomach infections, soothe an upset stomach, treat constipation and diarrhea, and help reduce bloating. The antibacterial effects also make it effective for warding off staph infections.

Back to the topic of inflammation, rosemary can reduce inflammation all over the body – including muscles, joints, and blood vessels. Because of this, people who suffer from inflammatory conditions such as high blood pressure, gout, arthritis, and physical injuries may find that rosemary helps reduce inflammation and ease their pain.

Consuming and Using Rosemary

Obviously, rosemary is most commonly consumed in food. Most kitchens have a little bottle of rosemary tucked away in a cupboard or spice rack. Rosemary is a generally well-liked herb that can be used in a wide variety of recipes, making it easy to incorporate into your diet. If you aren't fond of rosemary's taste or don't cook very often, you can also consume it in capsule form. Health food stores and online retailers carry these pills. Eating rosemary in your food or taking supplements is the best way to use rosemary to treat inflammation and stomach issues and improves cognitive function and memory. You can find rosemary tea at most supermarkets and drink it to soothe an upset stomach. Most health food stores also sell rosemary essential oil, which can be used for aromatherapy.

Growing Rosemary

Plant your rosemary seeds indoors, and do so about eight to ten weeks before the estimated date for the last spring frost. When the seedlings begin to grow, you can plant them outside or simply move the pot outdoors. Remember that rosemary needs plenty of sunlight. During the first few weeks, you'll need to water your rosemary regularly. It's a slow-growing plant, but once it starts really growing more, you won't need to water it as often. Simply touch the soil and make sure that it feels a little moist. Only water when the soil feels dry.

To make essential rosemary oil, cut a few sprigs of fresh rosemary. Remove the leaves from the stems and then wash them. Lay the leaves out to dry. After the leaves have dried, put them in a canning jar. Fill the canning jar with safflower or sunflower oil, or any other oil that has a very light scent. Make sure that

the leaves are completely submerged in the oil. Seal
the jar tightly and set it on a windowsill or someplace
where it will get sunlight. Let it sit for a week,
checking it often to make sure that condensation isn't
forming. If you do see some condensation, be sure to
open the jar and wipe it out. After a week has
passed, you can strain the oil and begin using it for
aromatherapy.

To make rosemary tea, pluck a few sprigs of
rosemary. Cut off the leaves and gently rinse them in
cold water. Allow the leaves to dry, and then crush
them very lightly. Steep the crushed leaves in hot
water for a few minutes, allowing them to sit in the
water until you achieve your desired flavor. Strain the
leaves and then drink the tea.

You can also simply cut rosemary leaves and store
them in a tightly sealed jar, and sprinkle them with
your favorite recipes. You can really enhance the
flavor of any soups, sauces, meats, and fish that you
cook by adding rosemary to them. You can also
make your own salad dressing by infusing fresh
rosemary in olive oil. This also makes a yummy
dipping sauce for bread and rolls.

Conclusion

I hope that you found this eBook to be informative and interesting to read. The goal of this eBook has been to show people that the herbs that grow in our garden, we drink in our tea, and have in our spice racks can play a role in improving our overall health. Many people think that there are a lot of complicated instructions that you have to follow to be healthy. The truth is that little modifications like drinking an herbal tea every day or practicing aromatherapy can have a big impact on how your body looks, feels, and functions. Many of the common ailments that you experience on a regular basis can be treated, prevented, and alleviated by consuming and inhaling these medicinal herbs. I challenge and invite you to examine your overall health and identify the aspects that could use improvement. Can any of these herbs help you? Chances are that they can.

Hopefully, this eBook has given you the knowledge you need to start taking care of your body holistically and making changes to live a healthier life. You don't always need prescription medication or an over the counter drug. Sometimes a tea, salve, oil, or natural supplement can be just as effective. My other hope for you is that this eBook is just one thing you'll read on your journey to learning more about natural wellness. Please, continue learning about herbs and their amazing healing capabilities. There are hundreds of medicinal herbs out there that are waiting for you to discover them!